Simple, Sensible, & Stress Free

Healthy Weight Management

"Seeds of Thoughts"

Therapeutic Hunger

Cracking the Code for Enjoying a Healthy Life and a Healthy Weight

Avnish Bhardwaz   and Yvette Maurice

Table of Contents

Acknowledgement

Writing these acknowledgements has been most pleasurable part of writing this book, as I can now express my appreciation to various influences for directly or indirectly shaping my life. I am very fortunate to have wonderful family, friends, elders, teachers, work colleagues and other people in society who have been a source of inspiration and support for me. I feel really blessed to have them all in my life, but there are too many to name here, so I will simply express my sincere gratitude and love.

When I started sharing my concepts with my family, friends and colleagues they showed immense interest and asked many questions. The complexity of their questions and the variations in their individual responses and requirements led me to realise the need for a book that will share the various concepts, ideas and suggestions of explaining the concept and process of Therapeutic Hunger.

I also got a phenomenal response to blogs on some of these topics as well as encouragement to write a book for the benefit of the many people struggling with questions, ideas or just in need of a spark to start the change in their lives.

I look forward to the new friendships and community this book creates. Thank you for being part of the journey.

Avnish Bhardwaz

Introduction

This book is written as a result of several years of observations, research, and experimentation. There have been many books covering various diets, super foods, exercises and magic techniques for weight loss and healthy living. Almost all of them prescribe very measured solutions, with the same techniques prescribed for everyone.

With Therapeutic Hunger, our objective is to cultivate the habits and build our senses for eating the right amount of food, breathing well and maintaining the right posture, all the time. We can do this by being aware about these things; starting with small deliberate actions and gradually getting to our objective of happy, healthy and harmonious living". Various ideas, practices, discussions and suggestions in this book will help you in achieving this objective with simple and easy means.

We are all individuals; we have different sizes, shapes, life styles and conditions. For this fact, we need to tailor individual solutions: what we eat, when we eat, how we eat. Similarly for exercise and other activities as well, we need to adjust ourselves according to our individual needs and capacity. As time and conditions change, we need to again adjust our eating, exercises and other activities– in order to enjoy good health and maintain a healthy body.

Be aware that food is only one of the many energy sources needed for good health. Our bodies need to have a fine balance of all life forces for physical, mental and emotional health and wellbeing. Understanding the 'right priority' of harmony and balance of various *factors will help us building 'right habits' and getting rid of ineffective behaviours.*

Our body, mind and emotional health are all interconnected. How each of these impacts on digestion and nutrition absorption also needs to be understood. We need to understand our individual needs and capacity and adjust our food intake, activities and relaxation accordingly. Only a good understanding of our bodies and how to balance our food intake with individual needs and capacity will lead us to live enjoyable and healthy lives.

Good Habits are formed through a very similar process that leads us to bad habits. Correcting these behaviours (whether good or bad habits) is a very similar process and can be done quite easily through understanding, courage and commitment. In this book, we will explain various topics and share stories of challenges and success. These stories will unravel the knots of every day issues and habits surrounding eating and hunger. Most of us can relate to some of the stories—celebratory eating, comfort eating, angry eating, and eating from boredom, "don't know why I am eating", and so on. This book will help us to create awareness and discover our own path, allowing us to make our own, best choices.

The chapters in this book will teach you to build up your senses so you can free yourself from old habits and create greater awareness for what to eat, when to eat and how much to eat.

Best Wishes!

Avnish Bhardwaz and Yvette Maurice

Disclaimer and Caution

The information provided in this book, and other reference materials are strictly suggestions only and are not in any manner given as a substitute for medical advice or direct guidance from a qualified health professional.

Always, in particular if you have a specific medical condition, consult your health care professional and obtain a full medical clearance before changing your eating habits or taking on any other exercise program. These suggestions strongly recommend careful, incremental and gradual changes in your eating and exercise program. At any time if you feel discomfort or pain, consult your healthcare professional. Not all practises are suitable for everyone. Consult your healthcare provider to discuss the changes you are going to make to your eating habits and exercises if you have any known medical conditions to determine what changes are most suitable for your particular case.

The authors, illustrators, editors, publishers and distributors assume no responsibility or liability for any injuries or losses that may result from practicing TH or any other exercise program. The author, editors, illustrators, publishers and distributors all make no representations or warranties with regards to the completeness or accuracy of information on this book, any linked websites, or other products represented herein.

Therapeutic Hunger
Manage your Hunger

Welcome to a Natural Way of Eating: with care, understanding and awareness.

Therapeutic Hunger: What is it?

Firstly, I would like to clarify the term "Therapeutic Hunger" (TH), to differentiate it from the hunger that is associated with problem issues like famine, poverty and eating disorders.

"Therapeutic Hunger" (TH) is the residual hunger that is left when we don't eat until our stomach is completely full. When we finish meals, and have eaten exactly the right quantity of food, we find that we don't feel full; there is still room in our stomach to properly process the food and make it ready for nutrients to be absorbed in intestines. This sweet hunger feeling is very therapeutic, as it helps optimise digestion, proper absorption of nutrients, and appropriate elimination of waste.

Your Hunger Helps the Organs to Work More Efficiently

In today's day and age, people fear hunger. They are constantly being told to eat every couple of hours, to never skip meals and to consume energy drinks and snacks between meals. In this way we are time bound for all these activities and never get to a point of feeling hungry. TH is a way to get your body's organs to work more efficiently by constantly providing signal to digest and absorb and keep functional space for proper digestion, absorption and elimination.

Our Organs Need a Space to Function and Digest food properly

Our body parts have evolved to work in such a way, so as to conserve energy; they will not perform any unnecessary task. So when there is a bountiful food supply, our organs don't need to digest food fully or extract nutrients most efficiently. Our abdomen is like a food processor; when it's filled over its natural limit it can't process food efficiently. It needs space to digest the food. There is a minimum and maximum level which is based on individual capacity and it works best at optimum capacity – we have called it TH. Both extreme dieting and over eating negatively impact digestion and our health.

Diagram below captures TH between two extremes of starvation and over eating.

Over Eating

Optimum Zone

Therapeutic Hunger

Normal Hunger

Extreme Dieting/Starvation

The Secret to Better Living is Avoiding Over-Eating

If we make it a habit to always eat just the amount of food, so as to leave some "Therapeutic Hunger" (TH), this will improve our health and control our weight by digesting food, and better absorbing nutrients. Practising TH may seem hard in the beginning, but later it will feel good: like a sweet hunger. This remaining hunger is actually a very good feeling, as one can enjoy the various tastes of the food; digest the food well and gain other benefits of good health. Make your start with small steps and gradually move towards your goal of a healthy, happy and harmonious life.

The Toxic Modern Lifestyle

In today's day and age, we are used to eating at fixed times and in fixed amounts. We tend to have a routine for breakfast, lunch and dinner. Our serving sizes are also more or less fixed, as suggested in the food recipes, or by the packets that our processed food comes in. Even the most flexible weight loss programs suggest the size of meals you should eat, irrespective of your hunger needs.

TH prescribes a new way of eating: instead of sticking to the habit of eating at fixed times, and in fixed quantities, we need to build up our senses to eat only when we are hungry and we need to focus on the right amount of food for our individual needs. Generations past have spread the "waste not, want not" mantra. Certainly, the desire not to waste food is an admirable one, but remember it is better to "waste" food on the plate than to let it waste inside your body and cause damage to your health.

Alcohol, Caffeine and Other Stimulants

Dependence on stimulating agents like coffee, tea, alcohol, tobacco and other substances doesn't help us, and can actually hinder our progress. These substances mask our senses and we can slowly lose control of our ability to taste, smell and sense when we are full and satiated (satisfied). People who practise TH are encouraged to drink water instead of soft drinks, and gradually reduce their dependence on stimulants that give short term relief, but that desensitise our senses.

The Therapeutic Hunger Handbook

This handbook will be your guide to eating with greater awareness, choosing the correct foods that you need to eat. You will learn how to be guided by your inner wisdom and intuition to let you know when to stop. Learning more about your digestion and metabolism will pay huge dividends in your physical and mental health and wellbeing.

Remember: It is better to waste food on the plate, than waste it in our body and damage our health.

Good luck. Let us begin our journey.

It is TRUE: "Eat breakfast like a king, lunch like a prince and dinner like a college kid with a maxed out charge card" - conditions apply.

Terms and Conditions: King, Prince and Kid all should practice Therapeutic Hunger, all the time, according to their individual needs and capacity.

Mindful Eating:

Most of time, we are multitasking while eating: Rather than focusing our full attention on the task at hand, we might be having business meetings, reading something, watching TV or catching up with family. All these activities are important, no doubt about it. However, if we think with a calm mind, we realise that eating well and living a healthy life are just as important.

Multitasking while eating can be harmful to our health

Most of us are time poor, these days; we need to do lot of tasks. However, if we are low on energy, unsteady in our mind, and suffer from health issues – does it actually help to try to get more done by multitasking? Ask yourself this question, and the answer seems obvious: No.

Whatever your level of health; if you spare some to eat well, properly, and mindfully - you are likely to work more efficiently and get more done in the remaining time. You will be more productive and achieve more, in less time and might even have spare time for further improvements.

Mindfulness when eating is Important

When we eat, it is imperative to think about the food, the ingredients, and the taste in every bite we take. Pay attention to food breaking down, and then to all the organs in the body which become fully engaged in its digestion as the nutrients transfer to the cells. While you concentrate on this, be thankful, and aim to make the process even better and more efficient, by being present with it. Once you commit to mindful eating, your organs will appreciate the attention and reward you with more nutrition, energy and health.

Scientific studies have also indicated that there is improved blood flow to the digestive organs when we pay attention to the food we are eating and do not have other distractions around us at that time.

Think about this: Imagine that your organs are like naughty children, if you pay attention to them they remain disciplined and work well, but the moment you take your attention away they start misbehaving and stop working to their greatest efficiency.

Mind, Body and Senses: Working in Harmony

Mindful eating improves our health. Our mind and senses begin to work in harmony and this provides us with immense paybacks with better health and a calmer mind. If we are freed from this unconscious habitual living, if we practise mindfulness, slowly but surely, we are pleasantly surprised, and we start to see that all our mental excuses for keeping old patterns of eating no longer hold up.

Know your metabolic system

Getting in touch with your metabolic system is an exercise and learning process that we all can enjoy. It is a gastronomic enlightening delight when you feel your stomach smiling back at you.

Remember: Mindful eating will accomplish - More Energy, Proper Weight, and Better Health

Understand Digestion:

Just like a well-cooked recipe needs a delicate balance of ingredients, water and fire (heat). Digestion also needs all these three elements.

Choose your food carefully: *Include a mix of proteins, carbohydrates, vitamins, fats and other minerals.*

Select the proper drink: *If done with care, this will enhance the taste, improve digestion and also might have ingredients in liquid form.*

Maintain the "Fire in the belly": *Hunger is this element that signals organs of the digestive track to perform effectively.*

What is the "Fire in the Belly"?

The first two elements of this mix (food and drink) are understood well by most of us, but the term 'fire in the belly' is used only in expressions, and does not usually refer to the internal digestive process. However, it is this fire in the belly that allows us to get the balance right for correct, efficient digestion of our food. Just as we need the right amount of tension and tuning for the various strings of a guitar to properly produce the musical notes, our bodies also need to require the fine tuning of the fire in the belly, to correctly produce effective digestion. Too much or too little of this "fire" will result in unpleasant sounds and feelings in the gut and belly. In summary, we need food, drink and fire in the right balance to digest food for good eating, better feeling and excellent health.

The Equation of Good Health

By paying attention to what we eat, when we eat and how we eat through "Mindful Eating", we can begin to build our senses to learn to recognise and achieve this balance of food, drink and fire. In order to do this, we need to pay attention to our body and to our feelings. If we make this a habit, it will serve us well throughout our lives, achieving good health and a happy life

Digestion Equation:

Total Digestion=Sum of Digestion of each bite of food eaten

OR,   Total Digestion=$\int A\,(1-nX)$

A is the average digestion of each bite of food.

n is the number of bites, X is the incrementally reduced hunger from each bite we eat

The purpose of showing this mathematical equation is to explain that the first bite we eat will have the maximum amount of digestion, as our hunger is highest at that time. As our hunger reduces with each subsequent bite, our body will take longer to digest bites of the same food. Once our hunger is completely gone, our digestion will slow down significantly.

Some Tips:

- *Keep a level of "Therapeutic Hunger", in order to maintain the digestive fire burning, or the "fire in the belly".*
- *Eat slowly if possible. Make time in your day to allow yourself to be more productive. This is turn gives you even more free time later to do more activities.*
- *Take a break. It allows your senses to send the correct signals to your brain about the amount of food your body needs. Normally, when we eat until our stomachs are full, we have already over-eaten, as there is often a delay from our senses to register the amount of food we eaten. By taking a break we allow the brain to register the amount of food consumed and how much more we need to eat.*

Remember: listen to the body and let it choose what it needs to eat and how much.

Eat More or Less

Some people relate eating 'more' with receiving greater nutrients or more energy in the body. This may be true as long as we are able to digest the food well and absorb the nutrients. Under the TH level, this will be the case. Overeating on the other hand has a damaging effect on our health.

Waste not, want not?

Some people don't like wasting food on the plate, in fact, many people have been taught this since childhood. In its essence, it is an admirable thought, but only effective if we have the right amount of food on our plate, which is very difficult at certain times and under certain conditions. It is better to waste the food on the plate, instead of wasting it inside our body, causing discomfort and also the potential to damage our health.

The "detoxing" fad

Similarly, extreme dieting, fasting and detox techniques should be handled carefully, as the effects of these can be quite negative on our health and wellbeing. Our body struggles with any sudden changes, but it adapts well when the changes are gradual. We can use this to our advantage for forming good healthy habits.

More food does not equal more energy

Eating more doesn't necessarily mean more energy in the long run. It might seem so for a short while, but we should be aware of the long term impact on our health and wellbeing. The key to good health is in *eating the right amount of food that our bodies can digest and getting all the nutrients our organs can absorb. We can learn these habits only by building our intuitive powers and paying attention to our body's signals.*

Gradually build your intuition to know, the right amount of food for your individual needs and capacity. Try squeezing your stomach towards your spine, and when you feel it is becoming slightly harder, this might help you to determine the time to slow, pause or stop eating. This might be just one of several signals to build your intuition and habit of eating the right amount of food.

We all have an individual, unique metabolism; a good diet that is self-taught is the best and most effective diet of them all. It is so important to understand which foods agree with us and which ones do not suit our bodies as much.

Remember: Feed the fluttering, flapping butterflies in your stomach- don't kill them by squeezing too much food in, leave some space to keep the butterflies alive and fluttering for good health!

Basal Metabolic Rate (BMR):

Today we eat with no awareness

Everybody has different nutritional needs. These vary with age, gender, height, level of activity and even ethnicity. Every human body burns energy all day and night. The body gets its energy from food, though its calories/kilojoules. Food is converted to energy by the muscles and tissues, and it is this energy which keeps them running.

Our organs and tissues need energy to keep them running; pumping our blood around our bodies all day and night. We are constantly burning the food we eat as fuel, so this needs to be replaced, which is who we get hungry. Even if a body is lying down in bed all day, it still uses up energy, and therefore calories and fuel.

TH helps you tune into your body's energy needs

Because we all have different energy needs, practising TH will help you to learn to hear the cues your body is giving you. This will prevent you from overeating, if you practise correctly. You will not need to count calories or control portion sizes, based on numbers and measures.

BMR or Basal Metabolic Rate

Men burn more calories than women; young people burn more calories than older people, and active people burn more than inactive people. You own body burned more energy at age 20 than it will (or did) at age 60. The amount of energy you burn each day can be calculated, based on your gender, age and activity level.

Your BMR can be worked out with the use of online calculators (simply type "BMR calculator imperial/metric" into your search engine).

You are not a number: listen to your body

We all have different energy needs, and studies have indicated that some people with the same statistics in age, gender and activity level still have different nutritional and energy needs. That is why it is so essential to pay attention to the cues your body is giving you. That's why learning to recognise Therapeutic Hunger is so essential. BMR explains part of the picture, but it is not the full story.

How to choose right foods for right digestion

Most foods can be segmented into three main categories.

1. **Harmonious:** *Easy to digest and absorb. Right balance of nutrients as per the needs of physical and mental activity.*
2. **Energising:** *Slightly harder to digest and gradually increase energy in the body, increase warmth and activity.*
3. **Sluggish:** *Hardest to digest, quick burst of energy and can make the body lazy in the long run.*

Harmonious foods *are foods such as lightly steamed vegetables, fruits, boiled fish etc. These foods are easy to digest, but should still only be consumed in moderate quantities. These are the most appropriate types of food that are suitable for people with a moderate level of activity.*

Energising foods *are needed when we have a high level of physical activity, and when our body needs the additional energy. Spicy foods* and stir fried foods vegetables and moderate quantities of food fall in this category.

Sluggish Foods provide a quick burst of energy and hard to digest. Deep fried foods, stimulants and intoxicants fall in this category. Such foods have a detrimental effect on the body and the senses, thus leading to poor health.

It is therefore necessary to understand the types of foods we need to suit our individual needs and capacity. We should adjust what we **need** to eat based on our activity level, which can vary from day to day, season to season. We should eat when we are hungry and eat just enough so as to still have little bit of hunger left, the "butterflies" we spoke about in the last section.

And what about calories?

Many health practitioners talk about monitoring calories, advising their clients to adjust the amount of exercise they need to do to compensate for any additional calories consumed. While on the surface this seems like a good idea, it is a faulty logic. To suggest exercise as a compensation for incorrect nutrition is ineffective. This way we get stuck on a rollercoaster; the damage is done and the bad habits are formed It is much better to keep control of what to eat in first place and cultivate the right habits according to individual needs. Why eat more if we just have to burn it later? Eat according to individual needs and capacity. Eat the right food in the right quantity that we can easily digest and absorb for growth, regeneration and healing.

The importance of an individual diet

Creating your own diet should be an adventure towards discovering the foods that your body has an affinity with. This should be seen as a journey of self-discovery as you work out the myths and secrets of your own internal organs. No expert knows your conditions, needs and capacity. Their advice is based on their experiences and knowledge. Knowing which foods to eat, knowing when to eat and how to eat should not be the knowledge of the select few. One can use their advice as a guide, although ultimately without our own stomach participating, this advice becomes useless and fruitless.

Choosing the right foods in the correct quantities will not only improve your physical health, it will also help you improve your mental health and to handle stress more effectively.

Remember: Eat hard to digest foods first, when the hunger is its peak and stomach can process the most.

Breathe well to feel well

In addition to the food we eat, to sustain life, there are many other energy sources. Some of these are air we breathe, sun light and other cosmic life forces that we perhaps don't understand much at the moment. Food it seems much over rated source for nourishing life and source of energy. Don't ignore other forces that sustain life – breathing, sun, and other cosmic energies. When we eat less, body will draw more from other life forces.

Breath: The Source of Life

Breathing is one of the most important activities for nourishing life – it is first thing we do as we are born and it is the last thing we will do as we leave this world. We can live without food for several days, but can't live without breathing even for few minutes. The way we breathe also affects the way we feel about ourselves and live our lives – and other way around is also true. Under stress the breath is shallow and fast. Similarly through slow and deep breathing we can increase relaxation and better control on our lives. We can also significantly increase our physical energy levels and mental clarity through proper breathing. Yet we pay so little attention to breathing and take it for granted as an unconscious mechanism for life sustenance.

Breathing allows us to balance our Life Force

The way we breathe affects our state of mind, energy level, emotional feeling and even our posture. In yoga, the breath is known as prana (or "life force") that can be used to find a balance between the body-mind. Unlike other bodily functions, the breath is easily used to communicate between these systems, which give us an excellent tool to help facilitate positive change. It is the only bodily function that we do both voluntarily and involuntarily. We can consciously use breathing to influence the involuntary (sympathetic nervous system) that regulates blood pressure, heart rate, circulation, digestion and many other bodily functions. Breathing exercises can act as a bridge into those functions of the body of which we generally do not have conscious control.

- Slow, deep, regular and calm breathing will relax your body and significantly improve your health & wellbeing.
- Rapid, short and quick breathing for few seconds can increase your energy level.

Training the Breathing Process:

Breathing can be trained for both positive and negative influences on our health. Chronic stress leads to decreased range of motion of the chest. Due to rapid, shallower breathing, the chest does not expand as much as it would with slower deeper breaths, and much of the air exchange occurs at the top of the lung. This results in "upper chest" breathing. Upper chest breathing is inefficient because the greatest amount of blood flow occurs in the lower part of the lungs; areas that have limited air expansion in chest breathers due to compression near the abdominal area. Rapid, shallow, upper chest breathing results in less oxygen transfer to the blood and subsequent poor delivery of nutrients to the tissues. The good news is that we can train the body to improve its breathing technique. With regular practice we will breathe from the abdomen most of the time, even while asleep. We can also do it ourselves by paying attention and self-study on multiple internet resources. Choose the one most suitable for individual needs and we can feel the benefits.

Remember: gradually improve breath awareness and get into good habits without trying too hard, too fast or too much

Right Posture & Spinal Health is vital for over all wellbeing.

At first, the title of this chapter may seem odd: what does spinal health have to do with good eating and digestion? In reality it is an important link in the complex chain of health and wellbeing.

It is true; when you see a healthy person you will also find a strong spine. The reverse is also generally true: when you see a healthy spine – you will find a healthy person.

When we have poor posture our internal organs are compressed against each other. All this compression can put pressure on the organs and cause digestive problems. By having good posture, we keep things nice and open for our intestines to do their work. A good posture, healthy spine allows more space for our organs to function properly. When spine is erect, body posture is good, we breathe better through diaphragm. Digestion efficiency is also increased when body organs aren't compress against each other, and have happy space to function normally.

A strengthened spine and correct posture will increase our energy levels. This will also reduce our dependence on food for our energy needs and require us to eat less food. Spinal twist exercises also improve digestion, add flexibility to the spine, Cleanse our Organs and Align the Spine for improved posture.

We can do twists from all kinds of positions: seated, standing, lying with legs bent, lying with legs straight, squatting and kneeling. Choose the one most comfortable and gradually build up the pace, as the spine alignment and strength improves. We should always be mindful of our own body. Never do anything that causes a sharp, destructive pain, especially in the back. The integrity is self-observation and learning from that observation, not pushing our body into any pain. Conscious breathing is far more important than how deep the twist goes

Remember: "You are as young as the agility of your spine"

Suggested Exercises

To be done with

Simplicity and Ease

Meditation

Meditation helps to control mental distractions, enhance clarity of thought and heightens awareness. The best way is to start from whatever your current level of experience is and to gradually increase your capacity to relax and concentrate. I have seen many advertisements for meditation workshops and training. I am not sure how anyone can teach meditation; one of the great things about meditation is that there's no "right" way to do it. Yes, techniques to distract and relax can be shared, but that might not be true meditation with lasting effects.

Meditation is meant to slow down movement of thoughts and relax the mind. Movement of thoughts are created by bondages such as desires, fears, cravings, anxieties, jealousy, etc. We really need to work to free ourselves from these bondages, create our own solutions that are tailored to suit our own individual needs. While soothing sounds, sweet incenses and a gentle breeze can help provide good a environment, we still need to calm the mind for lasting liberation and peace.

To begin meditation sit in a comfortable and relaxed position with a straight back, and concentrate on your breath. Take a deep breath gently through the nose, exhale like a soft sigh through the mouth. Imagine you have a shield around you, and no one can intrude through this shield into your space. This is your space - safe, secure and calm. Repeat this breathing till your mind has calmed down. When you are settled and relaxed continue to the next stage, concentrating on the sound and feel of your breathing. Focus on the sound of your inhalation and the soft, relaxing exhalation.

Concentrate and feel the breath of life flow through your body, feel your lungs naturally expand, the movement resembling the gentle ebb and flow below the oceans waves. Focus on the rise and fall of your chest, feel the gentle breath come and go, taking with it all your tensions as you settle into your calm and inner being where you can hear the pulse of your heart. Continue focused on your deep breathing, and feel yourself slowing down into the depth of the calm within, and be aware of it. You are now completely in tune with your inner self and the outside world ceases to exist for the while.

Remember: Calmness, Contentment and Control deliver lasting peace

Abdominal Breathing Technique

The diaphragm is the large muscle that separates our chest and our abdomen. When we move this muscle our breathing is very efficient, as we can steadily expand and contract our chest cavity. If we breathe only from the upper chest (as most of us do) we only use the upper chest cavity for breathing in and out.

The following exercise can help rebuild the habit for deeper abdominal breathing:

- *Place one hand on your chest and the other on your abdomen. When you take a deep breath in, the hand on the abdomen should rise higher than the one on the chest. This insures that the diaphragm is pulling air into the base of the lungs.*
- *When inhaling through the nose, take a slow deep breath in through your nostrils imagine that you are sucking in all the air in the room and hold it for a count of seven.*
- *Slowly exhale through your mouth for a count of eight. As all the air is released with relaxation, gently contract your abdominal muscles to completely remove the remaining air from the lungs. It is important to remember that we enhance respiration not just by inhaling more air but also by completely exhaling it.*

Repeat the cycle five more times for a total of 10 deep breaths and try to breathe at a rate of one breath every 10 seconds. At this rate, 6 breathe per minute, our heart rate variability increases, and this is also good for cardiac health.

Pelvic Floor Exercises:

Intense contraction and release of the pelvic floor muscles will help you strengthen these muscles to slowly gain better control. This will also improve your posture, and to create more space for better breathing and digestion. Moolbandha in Yoga terminology and Keigel Technique are some of the exercises that strengthen the pelvic floor muscles.

Squatting:

This is a lost art. These days we spend long hours sitting on chairs in the office or at home. The posture we adopt while sitting on a chair often compresses our organs and slows down our digestion. Squatting, on the other hand, stretches our muscles and aids our digestion.

Butterfly Pose

Caution: Do not this pose attempt if experiencing any knee problems.

This is a pose that improves our flexibility in the hip area. It is a very calming and light exercise that will also improve posture and improve health. Search for the butterfly asana on the internet.

Here is simple step-by-step guide:

- *First sit comfortably on a mat to do this pose.*
- *Then bend both knees, and move legs so that the feet, the soles and heels touch. Bring heels as close to the pelvic region as possible.*
- *Then reach out and hold the toes. Move knees like the wings of a butterfly, which means that they should be moved up and down.*
- *While doing this, make sure to keep the back straight.*
- *After performing the butterfly pose, unfold legs and straighten them. Shake them slightly and then relax.*

Benefits

This asana has several health benefits:

- *It increases flexibility of the hip joints.*
- *It increases the blood circulation in the legs.*
- *It is known to bring relief from numbness of legs, cramps, and sciatica pain.*
- *This posture is known to be a mood enhancer and can be good for relieving stress.*
- *It is known to relieve the tension in the inner thigh muscles.*

- If exhausted after walking or standing for long hours, then try this posture.

Caution: Do not attempt if experiencing any knee problem.

Bellows Breathing: Energising Exercise

This is an energising breath and will boost your energy levels. It is a good substitute for coffee or tea needed to boost energy.

- Sit in a comfortable upright position with your spine straight. Keep your mouth closed, breathe in and out of your nose as fast as possible. To give an idea of how this is done, think of someone using a bicycle pump (bellows) to quickly pump up a tire. Inhalation and exhalation both should take equal amount of time.
- The rate of breathing is rapid with as many as 2-3 cycles of inhalation/exhalation per second.
- While doing the exercise, you should feel some tension at the base of the neck, chest and abdomen. The muscles in these areas will increasingly become stronger the more this technique is practiced.
- Do not attempt this longer than 15 seconds when first starting. With practice, slowly increase the length of the exercise by 5 seconds each time. Do it as long as you are comfortably able, not exceeding one full minute.
- There is a risk for hyperventilation that can result in loss of consciousness if this exercise is practiced for a longer time in

the beginning. For this reason, it should be practiced in a safe place such as a bed or chair.

This exercise can be used each morning upon awakening or when an energy boost is needed during the day.

Health and Happiness

The body, mind and senses are closely linked. Cultivating the habit of happiness will improve your health and well-being. It is easier said than done, for sure. Taking small baby steps to get started can accomplish amazingly positive outcomes.

Once again the solutions are simple, similar and effective.

- Breathe well: at least 5 times a day bring your attention to your breath - slow, deep and rhythmic breathing.
- Several times a day make sure to check and correct your posture.
- Try light spinal twists a few times each day. Do this standing up or even when sitting on a chair.
- Abdominal exercise: When your stomach is empty, breathe out all air from the stomach and compress abdominal muscles. This is very useful exercise to do on an empty stomach in the morning.

A few important thoughts on essential ingredients for lasting happiness:

Most people these days tend to look for instant gratification. There are many short-term happiness solutions on offer, as we all know.

Examples of these include parties, concerts, holidays, running, exercising and even mediation. While some or most of these provide quick relief and even an impression of happiness, the effects don't last. Sometimes, the long-term side effects of some of these activities result in disappointment, frustration, loss and even depression.

What is true happiness?

So we ask ourselves, what would be needed for true happiness, and also to make it last? I will borrow a few words from the Sanskrit language to explain these points. The translation to English may not be exact, but here are the closest possible words. Sukha or happiness must contain all of the following three elements; Shanti (peace, calmness,), Santosha (contentment), and Sadbhavna (goodwill, respect, generosity).

All these elements peace, contentment and respect are also interrelated and interdependent. One cannot have true peace without being content with themselves and having respect for others. Similarly, it is also difficult to just be content and have no peace and generosity towards others.

- Shanti (peace, calmness, and quietude) will create mental clarity, to help in making the right choices in one's life.
- Santosha (contentment) will also help to accept and appreciate what one has and not be overly greedy or jealous.
    - "The greatest wealth is to live and be content with little." - Plato
- Sadbhavna (goodwill, respect, and generosity) will create a platform for growth of pleasure and happiness.

Once we have these three elements - peace, contentment and respect – we can experience true lasting happiness.

Relaxation and Sleep

Sound sleep and regular relaxation are very important for good health and wellbeing. There are many options for relaxation and we need to choose these very carefully.

***Thoughts on Sleep and Relaxation** We all know that relaxation calms us physically and mentally; it releases tension and it creates space in us, to organise ourselves and improve (if we understand and have willingness to take it forward).*

I will use an example to explain my point. Take a room fully cluttered with boxes. There is no space left and it is hard to find what you need, when you need it. What can you do to improve? First, you need to make space, so you can move the boxes around – categorise them by size, quality, usefulness, sensitivity, etc. After that you might be able to put smaller boxes inside larger ones and stack them properly in order. You might even find boxes that are not relevant to you and not needed any more. All of a sudden you find boxes organised and plenty of room created in the same space. Now it might even be easier than before to locate what you need and when you need it.

Our body and mind are similar as well. They need space to organise and function well. Relaxation is that process that creates the space, so that body and mind can organise better for higher performance and productivity. The space thus created allows us to access healing energies and improves health and well-being.

How do you choose to relax?

Relaxation can be done in many ways – holidays, parties, eating out, exercise, running, yoga, meditation, even drugs and alcohol. There are so many choices that people can avail of in order to relax themselves. We know that the choices we make will have their effects and consequences. I do not wish to go into each one, or justify which one is better than the other. The only point I would like to add here is that we need to think - while each relaxation method will help release tension, and create space - will I be able to take advantage of that space to organise my body and mind to stay organised in future?

Which is why it is only when you can create space and organise, the effects that you find they are sustainable and long-lasting. So choose the way you relax carefully and enjoy longer, and hopefully happy forever.

The importance of a good night's sleep

Sound sleep is necessary for good health and well-being. Getting enough quality sleep at the right time can help protect your mental health, physical health, quality of life, and safety. Sleep also supports healthy growth and maintenance. During deep sleep, our body releases the hormone that promotes normal growth and healing process. Sleep improves the immune system and also helps maintain a healthy balance of the hormones that make us feel hungry or full. It is thus necessary to cultivate good relaxation and sleeping habits.

A note on substances

Psychoactive substances, like alcohol, coffee and some energy drinks, act primarily upon the central nervous system and affect brain functions. These substances operate by temporarily affecting a person's neurochemistry, which in turn causes changes in a person's mood, cognition, perception and behaviour. While these substances are also used for recreation and therapeutic use, the impact of these on sleep and other mental functions should be kept mind.

Improve your control of abdominal muscles:

Abdominal Muscles Exercises (rapid abdominal muscle movements)

While standing straight bend slightly forward from the waist while keeping the back straight. This is like a hinge from the hips only and maintaining straight back. Make sure you get adequate support by resting your hands on your knees or just above so that the back is not strained. Please make sure the arms are straight.

This exercise is best done on an empty stomach; do this in the morning before breakfast or late evening before dinner. It can also be done during the day, 2-3 hours after any main meal, when we feel the stomach is not so full. Breathe in deeply, and after this, slowly exhale fully contracting the abdomen and lungs so that all the air is expelled. While holding breath in this position, contract or 'flap' your abdominal muscles in and out. Note that this should be done rapidly while holding the exhaled position WITHOUT inhaling. Do this as many times as possible and then take a slow, deep breath inside. This is one round of the practice.

In the beginning we may find that we have no control on the abdominal muscles and are unable to coordinate the flapping movement. These muscles must be slowly developed over time. Therefore, in the beginning do five such rounds, each of 20 flapping cycles are more than enough. This should gradually be built up to 150 inward-outward flapping cycles in each round.

We may say what it has to do with TH? Improved strength in abdominal muscles improves posture and breathing. In turn it will increase intake of life forces from nature, reduce dependence on food intake and improve overall health. It is also a good way to build our intuition to stop eating when we find it is becoming harder to squeeze your stomach towards our spine. While we are eating food, gently squeeze our stomach few times when we exhale breath. This exercise will help us to pay attention to breathing and good posture as well as give us a good indication to stop eating when it gets bit harder to squeeze your stomach during exhale.

Typical Obstacles

&

How to overcome them

How to overcome - Cravings for food

This is a common challenge faced by most people. Cravings are caused by uncontrollable movement of thoughts. Learning to control the mind is perhaps one of the most valuable things a person can do in his or her lifetime. However, it takes diligence, work and commitment; it will not happen instantaneously, there is no magic pill.

How do we gain control of the mind?

To gain control of your mind, and subsequently your cravings for food, like with other suggestions, your goal should be to take small baby steps. A good way to start would be to conduct a simple exercise on yourself, simply eat half of what you wish to eat to satisfy your carving (whether it's salt, sugar or fat) and simply choose to be aware of the effects. By learning to tune in and listen to our bodies, we learn to understand the simple cues our bodies are giving us to let us know information about our health, our satiety and our energy levels.

Another thing to remember is that it is important to leverage the short term energy you have gained to practice for more positive outcomes in the future. Build on your successes! For example, I used to drink 3 to 4 cups of coffee each day. With control over my cravings, I managed to use this technique to stop drinking coffee completely. When I analysed my actions, I realised that I was drinking coffee to allow myself "a break in the routine" and also to enhance my alertness.

How I changed my habit:

42

My coffee habit started out innocently enough; but it was a habit that was becoming a distraction. I overcame my cravings for coffee in the way I described above. When I was craving a coffee, I would make one, but rather than drink it unconsciously, I started by taking only 2 to 3 sips from each cup. The quick injection of energy I gained, I then used to breathe deeper and improve my posture. I found that this energised me more, and slowly moved me from the habit of coffee drinking to the habit of better breathing and improved posture. I used one habit to instil another.

A note on mental chatter:

In today's world, there is a lot of information that our brains have to process. Most of us find it hard to "shut down" or to "focus" on a task, as our minds are not quiet, but cluttered by many thoughts.

By becoming more aware, we learn to gain some control over our minds, so that we can effectively use the mind for its purpose. Once the mental chatter is slowed down, calmness prevails, and we can see and think clearer. This will free us from the bondages of craving and restoring peace to mind by gradually removing the disturbances.

Emotional Eating

Many people in ill health find themselves enslaved by emotional eating. It is challenging, but luckily it is also quite easy to overcome.

Negative emotions and losing control

Negative emotions like anger, panic, stress and anxiety have an adverse impact on our senses. As a result we lose control and awareness, which could lead to damaging outcomes and develop wrong habits. When we are aware, we are not reacting to the world around us. Emotions such as anger, panic, fear etc can cause us to lash out in ways that are not beneficial to us. How often do we lose our temper and think, "I can't believe I became that angry" once the source of our anger has gone away? This is because our emotions caused us to lose control. We became unaware of ourselves in that moment.

So what can be done about this?

How can we overcome our emotions, and therefore our emotional eating? If you would like to overcome emotional eating think about following:

*When you are walking along a path and come across a large hole in the ground in front of you, if you were to close your eyes you might not see the hole for a short time, until you opened your eyes again. To continue on our path, we either **need to** close the hole or walk around it to get to the other side. The same can be said for emotional eating.*

When we have a desire to eat for reasons other than hunger, our drive to eat is usually driven by an emotion. Comfort foods might provide short term relief from our feelings but cause far greater damage in the long run. A good technique is to distract yourself until your emotions settle down.

Instead of using food as a problem diversion, try some other alternatives.

- *Invent your own diversion technique that is calming and relaxing yet increases awareness of your surroundings*
- *If you are a religious person, your religious practices might help. Examples of this might be prayer or meditation.*
- *Ruby cube, counting beads*
- *Light stretching, like yoga and meditation could be very useful. You don't even need special instructions for these try simple ways... look for examples on the internet. Many exercises can be done from the comfort of your own home.*
- *Be creative, innovative , determined and courageous*
- *Be kind, polite and considerate*
- *Let go and forgive past actions (yours and others)*
- *Live in "the Now" and enjoy the Present*
- *Bring your attention to your breathing. Slow, deep and rhythmic breathing will quickly improve your mode.*
- *Pay attention to your posture and sit/stand correctly*
- *Listen to relaxing music*

How to Combat Emotional Eating:

The "Fast Food" culture

In this day and age, we consume food on the go. We skip breakfast, eat lunch at our desks, snack all day and eat dinner in front of the TV. We have lost the true pleasure that can be found in food.

Food provides our senses with sustenance. Food has texture, smell, taste, an appealing appearance, and sometimes even associated sounds, (a sizzling barbeque, a popping cork) and when we don't allow time for our senses to connect with the experience of eating, we may feel "cheated" or "denied" and feel as if we have not experienced the food at all.

So we eat more. We eat because we have not truly engaged our senses fully, and therefore we eat too much, seeking the experience that we set out to undertake physically.

How do we heighten our awareness while eating?

For this, we must return to the senses.

There is a reason that fine dining is done on a white table cloth, with clean plates and shiny cutlery or chopsticks. In order to experience food, we must return to the senses and make time to expertise the sensory experience of eating. To do this, we need to pay attention to the texture, taste, appearance, smell and even the sounds of our food.

Making time to eat

We need to make meal times an event. This is not always possible in our everyday, working lives. If we have a problem with emotional eating, eating too much or comfort eating, this is because we are not properly acknowledging our food. To acknowledge our food, we cannot simply stuff a sandwich in our mouths while we run for the train; we must take the time to fully experience the food. To do this we need to make meal times an event.

This does not mean that we need to allow an hour for each meal, always sitting down at a white table cloth. It does mean that when we eat we need to make sure we are not distracted by exterior elements. We need to make sure we are not reading, watching TV or working while we eat. We need to give ourselves 15 minutes to experience the food properly, enjoying its texture, taste, smell, sounds and appearance.

Set the place to eat

When you need to eat, leave your workspace, coffee table or bedroom. Eat at a space that is designed for eating, at a table, in the kitchen, or even outside under a tree. Choose a place that is different to where you were just working or living. Set you food on a proper plate when you can. Eat with cutlery or chopsticks when you can, as this slows us down and makes us eat more consciously.

Many little tastes keep your palate interested!

Have as many little tastes on the plate as you can, rather than one large portion of food that is all the same flavour. For example, it is easy to overeat if the only thing your senses have to experience is a large palate of cheesy macaroni pasta. Imagine the differences to the senses if you were to serve a small taste of the macaroni, with a crunchy salad and a small bowl of fresh vegetable soup. By having three small portions of food, rather than one large portion, your palate gets to receive more of a sensory experience, so it is satisfied more quickly and does not need to overeat.

Don't give food power that it does not have

One other thing to note with emotional eating is to make sure that you don't labour yourself with unrealistic expectations of what food can do for you. It cannot make you smarter, richer or more desirable. Food is a tool for your body to allow you to be the best you can be. Food is not your enemy; food is not your comfort. Food is a tool in your tool kit.

Do not let food become your master and your ruler. In order to have a happy relationship with food we need to master its use, and let it serve us in the fashion for which it was designed. By learning how to correctly listen to our body's cues, we will learn how to gain control of our eating.

What if I get hungry too quickly?

This is a question we often ask ourselves. Many people simply feel that if they eat small portions they may t get hungry again in one or two hours.

That is precisely the reason that no one can prescribe the portion size for you, or anyone else. One of the main teachings of Therapeutic Hunger is that it is up to us as individuals to determine our needs and capacity. Also our digestion of food varies depending on the type of food we have put into our bodies and our metabolism (capacity to digest).

It is thus necessary to understand the concepts discussed earlier in the book to fully understand how digestion works, the type of foods we should eat and their digestion efficiency, and to be aware of our body's needs and its capacity. Only us as individuals can decide our food intuitively, based on combination of these factors.

There are quite a few suggestions to consider so that we don't get hungry too quickly:

- *Decide what is "too quickly" for you: one hour, two hours, three hours*
- *Select the types of food you need accordingly and understand what is available*
- *Fill up in between meal times by drinking water or other suitable drinks such as herbal teas*
- *Consider mixing water into your other drinks such as fruit juice etc. this will reduce calories and gradually reduce any craving.*
- *Eat healthy snack in moderation and paying attention to your needs*
- *Gradually build your habits*

How to Develop Your Intuition:

What is intuition?

Intuition is one of our sensual faculties, as in "of the senses". We all know about our regular faculties: we use our five senses to gain information about the world. Likewise, we can use our "higher faculties" to gather information about our world, including the physical, spiritual and emotional. One of our higher faculties is our intuition.

We all have higher faculties that we can develop. Most people agree that there is such a thing as intuition, or the "gut feeling". It's when you get a hunch about something, an inner feeling that you can't explain through conscious thought.

Why is it important to develop?

This is a question I have been asking myself for years. Why should I be developing my intuition, and how does it differ from my conscious mind? When you are able to tune into your intuitive voice, you can get insights and extra information and your inner knowing can be developed. Our intellect is the part of us that seeks to rationalise things. Once we tune in to our intuition, we can tap into a higher cosmic force.

How can you develop your intuition?

Developing your intuition is like developing any muscle- you need to exercise your intuition to make it strong. We are all born with this faculty, and there are many ways of not just heightening your powers of intuition, but heightening your own faith in your intuition. Start to pay attention to any gut feelings you may get and ask yourself if it may be your intuition speaking to you. Here are some exercises that may help with developing intuition.

Meditation

By strengthening your level of concentration and focus, you can strengthen the mind. Practising meditation can be a good way to start.

Meditation can be developed as a necessary tool for life, like going to the gym. At first you might dislike going to the gym and getting on a treadmill – it's boring, repetitive and dull, but if you do half an hour of exercise every day for a month, you might start to see some of the benefit of it – and this encourages you to make it a part of your life.

If you want a strong mind, you need to learn how to concentrate. If you want to learn how to control your mind, then you should learn how to meditate. Some simple techniques below might help.

Breathing meditation

Concentrate on your breathing, and the intake and outtake of breath. Start with a meditation of 10 minutes a day, and build up from there. Sit in a comfortable position in a quiet space and concentrate on your breath, focusing only on that. If your mind wanders, then simply and gently return your attention to your breath.

Sweeping meditation

Sit in a comfortable position in a quiet space and relax yourself. Bring your attention to the crown of your head, and imagine relaxing your body in stages, relaxing each body part. Move through your chest, *arms, hands, trunk, legs and feet. Once you have completed this, begin at your feet and sweep back to your crown, relaxing each body part as you go. Repeat this exercise for 10 or 20 minutes.*

Choosing a line or lift

Try to develop your intuition in everyday life. When your phone rings; ask yourself who is on the line without looking at your caller ID. You can even try this one at lines in the supermarket – try to pick which line will get you to the counter first – it's not always the shortest one!

Use a different hand, walk a different way

Again, this is about developing a different pathway in your brain. A neural pathway connects one part of the nervous system with another via bunches of elongated neurons, serving to connect distant areas of the brain or nervous system. Some people believe that these pathways can be strengthened and developed by doing things with the opposite hand, for example, brushing your teeth with the other hand. You could also try taking a different route in your car or when on foot.

So why is it important to develop our intuition?

Developing our intuition lets us fully utilise our senses and gradually expands them. Life can be so confusing, but by learning to listen to the still space of quite within us, we can think better and experience more.

Extreme dieting, restricted diets, fasting and detox treatments

While don't want to dwell too much on these topics, it is necessary to mention a word of caution and bring attention to the risks that might be involved. It is always better to take small measured steps, monitor your progress, and gradually improve your health. Extreme measures might give quick short term results, but often not sustainable and involve high risks. Move with caution!

Do not shock your body

Sudden and drastic changes often result is imbalance that body could find hard to adjust. It could cause pain, headache, nausea, sleeplessness etc. Thus compounding the health problems even more or return to old habits.

Type 2 Diabetes:

Three years ago, I was diagnosed with Type 2 Diabetes. My doctor told me that I will have exercise more, adjust my life style and perhaps take medication. I was overweight and my BMI was high.

I tried to exercise but found it very challenging. This started my search for better and practical ways to improve health. I started with breathing exercises, gentle stretches (basic yoga – self-taught), and discovered Therapeutic Hunger. A gradual combined approach of all three: Breathing, gentle mindful exercises (for spinal health and good posture) and eating well (TH) has helped me overcome diabetes, get back into good weight and shape, feel energised and enjoy life. All these are now integrated in my day to day activities that I don't need to set a daily or weekly time aside. Plus I feel far more energetic, and much more productive. Any additional time I set aside for exercise is additional bonus, but not necessary when I have other pressing needs, I pay attention to breathing, right postures several times a day and keep Therapeutic Hunger all the time. It is almost effortless and automated response now.

Step by Step Guide

Building Good Habits: Step By Step Guide

Both good and bad habits are formed through a similar process. Habits can be easy changed by the following: "Think before You Act" strategy. It is not a matter of willpower or mental strength, or anything else.

Here are some tips; I can share towards building good eating habits:

1. *Make a commitment to eating well and to not eating too much.*
2. *Understand TH and visualise the future benefits*
3. *Every time you eat, think about TH*
4. *Enjoy the nutrients, and flavours of your food*
5. *Replace earlier habits with a new habit (Leaving TH)*
6. *Repeat it unit you get used to it (this might be 10 days to a month in most cases)*

You can also adopt these steps for forming other habits as well.

Practicing Therapeutic Hunger

This is step by step guide to practice TH, providing the steps that will allow you to make it a natural habit. In my own experience, and in the experiences of other people who are practicing TH now, it often takes about 10 days of paying attention to eating in moderation, for it to become easy and natural. After that it becomes quite easy and you find that your intuitive behaviour is to eat well and in the right amounts.

Attention should be paid to both the nutrients, and the amount of food as well as the food volume. Sometimes we might have to skip having a drink for 30 minutes or so after we eat, to ensure that the abdomen is not more than 75% full and has empty space to process the food properly.

This can be delayed for as little as a few minutes to up to 30 or 40 mins after eating our food. If the food you are eating is dry and you really do need to drink something along with it, make sure you only eat until your stomach is 75% full at a maximum.

10 Steps to good physical and mental health

1. *Remember Therapeutic Hunger each time you eat.*
2. *You can eat as many times as you like during the day, as long is your stomach is not more than 75% full.*
3. *Pay attention to your breathing: Slow, deep and rhythmic breathing should be practised few times a day.*
4. *Try abdominal breathing for a few minutes first thing in the morning and later again in the afternoon.*

5. *Practice* bellows *breathing, before meals when stomach is empty, to energise the body. This will also help to reduce your dependence on stimulants like coffee, tea, cola or other energy drinks*

6. *Correct your posture several times a day.*

7. *Build spinal agility and exercise spinal support muscles. Use gentle exercises.*

8. *Avoid drastic diet changes or exercises that can have adverse effects.*

9. *Keep your objective in mind and gradually build habits to accomplish it.*

10. *Eating well, breathing properly and keeping the right posture will help you achieve your heath back. Like most of us enjoyed back in our childhood.*

Website to information and FAQs:
http://www.positivehunger.com

Summary

A three-pronged approach is necessary to summarise the healthy habits discussed in this book:

- **Eat Properly**: *Right Food, Right Time and Right Quantity*
- **Breathe well:** *Slow, Deep and Rhythmic breathing-abdominal control*
- **Right Posture:** *Maintain good body posture – so the organs can function properly*

Keeping in the above 3 things in mind, slowly cultivate the habits and reap the rich rewards.

What will success look like?

- *Improved health*
- *Higher level of energy throughout the day*
- *Mental calmness*
- *Clearer thinking*
- *Living in harmony – with the world around us.*
- *Enjoying greater Health and Happiness*

Website to information and FAQs:

http://www.positivehunger.com

Authors:

Avnish Bhardwaz: *30+ years veteran in healthcare engineering, innovation and programs management. He has travelled around the world for work and leisure. Takes keen interest in various cultures, philosophies and people. Respects all religions and beliefs and follows what is relevant for a particular time, place and conditions. This book is a result of years of research, observations and experimentation. Sharing experiences and hoping to make this world a better place to live for everyone.*

Yvette Maurice *is a freelance journalist and copywriter with nearly two decades of media experience in radio, print, TV and online. She has previously worked for Southern Cross Austereo and Macquarie Media Network as an announcer, producer and promotions director. With a personal passion for health and fitness, Yvette enjoys learning about nutrition, new nutrition techniques, and about how to effectively manage our bodies for maximum health and wellbeing. In her spare time Yvette likes to read memoirs, cook vegetarian food and practise yoga.*